**Thank you for purchasing our book.
We hope you love it!**

Unlock the secrets to lasting weight loss with "5 Essential Steps to Permanent Weight Loss: Insights from a Fitness Insider." This transformative guide gives you expert knowledge and actionable strategies to achieve and maintain your ideal weight.

Copyrights©

Table Of Contents

Chapter 1: Understanding Permanent Weight Loss

The Importance of a Sustainable Approach

Sustainability in weight management is crucial for achieving lasting results, particularly for women navigating various life stages. As hormonal changes occur during menopause or pregnancy, the need for a balanced, sustainable approach becomes even more evident. This method emphasizes gradual changes and long-term habits rather than quick fixes or extreme diets that may lead only to short-term success. By prioritizing sustainable practices, women can foster a healthier relationship with food and exercise, ultimately leading to more effective weight management.

A sustainable approach encourages mindful eating, which helps individuals develop awareness of their hunger and fullness cues. This technique is particularly beneficial for busy professionals and new parents, who may find themselves eating on the go or in response to stress. By focusing on the quality of food consumed and savoring each bite, individuals can reduce the likelihood of emotional eating and make more conscious choices.

This strategy not only aids in weight loss but also contributes to overall well-being, making it easier to maintain a healthy lifestyle amidst life's demands.

Integrating fitness and nutrition is another pillar of sustainability in weight management. For fitness enthusiasts and athletes, having a tailored regimen that aligns with nutritional needs is essential. A balanced diet that supports physical activity enhances performance and promotes recovery, while a consistent workout routine helps build muscle and boost metabolism.

This synergy between diet and exercise creates a comprehensive framework for individuals at any stage of life, reinforcing the idea that sustainable weight management is not merely about calories in versus calories out but rather about creating a holistic lifestyle.

Building a support system can further enhance sustainability in weight loss efforts. Whether through friends, family, or online communities, having a network of like-minded individuals can provide motivation, accountability, and encouragement. Many women experience unique challenges related to weight management, and sharing experiences within a supportive group can foster resilience and commitment. This community aspect can be particularly beneficial for seniors and individuals with health conditions, offering both emotional support and practical advice tailored to specific challenges.

Lastly, the role of sleep cannot be overlooked in the pursuit of sustainable weight loss. Poor sleep patterns can disrupt metabolism and lead to increased cravings, making it more difficult to maintain a healthy weight. Prioritizing sleep is an integral part of a sustainable approach, ensuring that the body has the opportunity to rest, recover, and regulate hormones effectively. By understanding and implementing the principles of sustainability in both diet and lifestyle, individuals can achieve permanent weight loss and, more importantly, improve their overall health and quality of life.

Common Misconceptions About Weight Loss

One of the most pervasive misconceptions about weight loss is that it can be achieved through drastic calorie restriction. Many individuals believe that eating as little as possible will lead to quick results. However, this approach often backfires, leading to a slowed metabolism and potential nutritional deficiencies. Sustainable weight loss relies on a balanced intake of nutrients that support the body's needs while creating a moderate caloric deficit. Instead of extreme dieting, focusing on portion control and nutrient-dense foods can foster healthier habits that are easier to maintain over time.

Another common myth is that all carbohydrates are bad for weight loss. This belief can lead to unnecessary fear of foods like fruits, whole grains, and legumes, which are essential for a well-rounded diet. Carbohydrates are the body's primary energy source, and when chosen wisely, they can play a significant role in weight management. Emphasizing complex carbohydrates over refined sugars and processed foods can help maintain energy levels while supporting weight loss goals. Understanding the difference between healthy and unhealthy carbs is crucial for sustainable eating practices.

Many people also think that exercise alone is sufficient for weight loss, overlooking the critical role of nutrition. While physical activity is important for burning calories and maintaining muscle mass, it cannot compensate for poor dietary choices. A successful weight loss strategy integrates both exercise and mindful eating. This balanced approach ensures that individuals not only burn calories through workouts but also make informed decisions about their food intake, which is vital for achieving and maintaining a healthy weight in the long term.

Additionally, there is a misconception that weight loss is a linear journey, where consistent progress is guaranteed. In reality, weight loss can fluctuate and be influenced by various factors such as hormonal changes, stress levels, and lifestyle shifts. Understanding that setbacks are normal can prevent discouragement and promote resilience. Emphasizing a holistic view of health rather than just the number on the scale encourages individuals to celebrate non-scale victories and recognize the broader benefits of their efforts.

Finally, many believe that weight loss is a one-size-fits-all process. Each person has unique needs based on their age, gender, health status, and lifestyle. Tailoring weight loss strategies to fit individual circumstances is essential for long-term success. This customization might include adjusting meal plans, workout routines, and even mindset approaches to better align with personal goals and preferences. Recognizing and embracing these individual differences can lead to more effective and sustainable weight management solutions.

The Role of Mindset in Achieving Goals

Achieving weight loss goals is not solely a matter of dietary choices or exercise routines; it fundamentally hinges on the mindset you cultivate throughout the journey. Mindset serves as the internal compass that guides your decisions, influences your behaviors, and shapes your resilience in the face of challenges. For women navigating various life stages, such as pregnancy or menopause, developing a positive and growth-oriented mindset becomes particularly vital. By adopting an attitude that embraces change and promotes self-compassion, individuals can lay a stronger foundation for sustainable weight management.

A growth mindset encourages individuals to view setbacks as opportunities for learning rather than insurmountable obstacles. This perspective is crucial in weight management, where progress is rarely linear. The ability to reframe failures—such as a missed workout or an indulgent meal—as learning experiences fosters resilience and keeps motivation intact. Women, especially, may find themselves facing unique challenges during different life stages, and understanding that these moments do not define their overall journey can empower them to persist and adjust their strategies accordingly.

Additionally, cultivating a mindful approach to eating and exercising can significantly enhance the weight loss experience. Mindful eating techniques encourage individuals to pay attention to their hunger cues and emotional triggers, promoting a healthier relationship with food. This awareness can mitigate emotional eating, a common hurdle that many face. When women learn to listen to their bodies and appreciate the experience of eating, they are more likely to make choices that align with their long-term health goals, thereby reinforcing a positive mindset toward weight loss.

Integrating fitness and nutrition is another critical aspect influenced by mindset. Embracing the belief that exercise can be enjoyable rather than a chore can lead to greater consistency and adherence to fitness routines. Finding activities that resonate with personal interests can transform the approach to physical activity from a requirement into a rewarding experience. As women explore different workout options, they not only enhance their physical health but also cultivate a mindset that celebrates movement as a vital part of life's joy.

In conclusion, the role of mindset in achieving weight loss goals cannot be overstated. A positive and adaptable mindset fosters resilience, encourages mindful eating, and promotes a joyful approach to fitness. As women embark on their weight management journeys, embracing this internal shift can result in more sustainable and fulfilling outcomes. By focusing on mindset alongside practical strategies, individuals can navigate the complexities of weight loss with greater confidence and success, ultimately leading to lasting change.

Chapter 2: Step One - Setting Realistic Goals

Defining Your Weight Loss Journey

Defining your weight loss journey is a crucial first step in achieving lasting results. Each individual's path is unique, shaped by personal goals, lifestyle, and circumstances. For women navigating various life stages such as pregnancy or menopause, understanding how these changes affect their bodies and metabolism is essential. Recognizing that weight loss is not a one-size-fits-all approach allows for the creation of a tailored plan that considers these nuances. This personalized perspective is key to maintaining motivation and commitment throughout the process.

To effectively define your weight loss journey, begin by setting clear, attainable goals. These goals should be specific, measurable, and time-bound, allowing you to track progress and adjust your strategies as needed. For busy professionals or new parents, integrating realistic objectives that fit into an already hectic schedule can make all the difference. By focusing on incremental changes rather than drastic transformations, individuals can cultivate habits that lead to sustainable weight loss over time.

Mindful eating is another essential component of this journey. Developing an awareness of hunger cues and emotional triggers can help mitigate the effects of stress and emotional eating, a common challenge for many. Practicing mindfulness involves not just what you eat but how you eat, encouraging you to savor meals and recognize when you are satisfied. This practice fosters a healthier relationship with food, making it easier to adhere to your weight loss plan and avoid the pitfalls of restrictive dieting.

Incorporating a balanced fitness regimen alongside nutrition is also vital for long-term success. Whether you're an athlete or a health-conscious individual, finding an activity you enjoy enhances adherence to a workout routine. Home workouts can be particularly beneficial for those with limited time, providing flexibility without sacrificing effectiveness. Combining strength training with cardiovascular exercises can boost metabolism and promote fat loss, leading to a more toned physique.

Lastly, building a support system is fundamental in defining and maintaining your weight loss journey. Surrounding yourself with like-minded individuals, whether through friends, family, or support groups, can provide encouragement and accountability. Sharing experiences and challenges fosters a sense of community, making the journey less isolating. Engaging with professionals, such as nutritionists or personal trainers, can also offer valuable insights tailored to your specific needs, further enhancing your path toward permanent weight loss.

SMART Goals for Lasting Change

Setting SMART goals is essential for achieving lasting change in weight management. The acronym SMART stands for Specific, Measurable, Achievable, Relevant, and Time-bound. By incorporating these principles into your weight loss journey, you can create a clear roadmap that guides your efforts and helps you maintain focus. This approach is particularly beneficial for women navigating different life stages, busy professionals, and individuals facing unique challenges. When your goals are well-defined, you are more likely to stay motivated and committed.

Specificity is crucial when defining your weight loss goals. Instead of stating a vague intention to "lose weight," articulate exactly how much you want to lose and the timeframe in which you aim to achieve it. For example, you might set a goal to lose 10 pounds in three months. This clarity allows you to develop targeted strategies, such as meal planning and incorporating exercise into your daily routine. The more specific your goal, the easier it becomes to design actionable steps that align with your desired outcome.

Measurable goals allow you to track your progress effectively. Instead of focusing solely on the end result, break your overall goal into smaller milestones. For instance, aim to lose one to two pounds per week, which can be monitored through weekly weigh-ins or body measurements. This measurable approach fosters accountability and encourages you to celebrate small victories along the way. By recognizing these achievements, you reinforce positive behaviors and maintain motivation throughout your weight loss journey.

Achievability is a critical aspect of goal-setting that ensures your objectives are realistic. Setting overly ambitious targets can lead to frustration and disappointment. Assess your current lifestyle, commitments, and any potential obstacles that may arise. For example, if you are a busy professional or a new parent, consider how much time you can realistically dedicate to exercise and meal preparation. Setting achievable goals allows you to progress steadily, making it more likely that you will sustain your efforts over the long term.

Relevance and time-bound criteria round out the SMART framework. Ensure that your goals align with your personal values and lifestyle. For instance, if you are focusing on health due to a specific medical condition, your goal should directly reflect that priority. Additionally, establishing a clear deadline for your goals fosters a sense of urgency and keeps you focused. By integrating the SMART criteria into your weight loss strategy, you create a sustainable plan that accommodates your unique circumstances, ultimately leading to lasting change.

Tracking Progress Effectively

Tracking progress effectively is a critical aspect of any weight loss journey, particularly for women navigating various life stages. Understanding how to monitor changes in weight, body composition, and overall health enables individuals to make informed decisions about their diet and exercise routines. This process involves more than just stepping on a scale; it requires a multifaceted approach that incorporates different methods of tracking, including measurements, food diaries, and fitness apps. By employing these tools, individuals can gain a clearer picture of their progress and identify areas that may need adjustment.

One effective method of tracking progress is through regular measurements of body composition. Instead of solely relying on weight, which can fluctuate due to various factors such as water retention or hormonal changes, women can measure their waist, hips, and other key areas. Keeping a record of these measurements over time can provide insight into fat loss and muscle gain, offering a more comprehensive understanding of one's body changes. This approach is particularly beneficial during life stages like menopause, when hormonal shifts can impact weight distribution and metabolism.

In addition to physical measurements, maintaining a food diary can be an invaluable tool for tracking eating habits. Writing down everything consumed throughout the day not only increases awareness of food choices but also helps identify patterns that may lead to emotional or mindless eating. By reviewing this diary regularly, individuals can pinpoint high-calorie snacks or meals that do not contribute to their nutritional goals. This practice fosters accountability and encourages mindful eating, which is essential for sustainable weight management.

Fitness apps can also play a significant role in tracking progress. Many of these applications allow users to log workouts, monitor daily activity levels, and track nutritional intake. By utilizing these tools, individuals can set specific goals, receive reminders, and gain insights into their daily habits. This digital tracking can be particularly useful for busy professionals or new parents who may struggle to find time for traditional methods of monitoring their progress. The convenience of technology allows for more consistent tracking, which is essential for long-term success.

Lastly, building a support system can enhance the effectiveness of tracking progress. Sharing goals and updates with friends, family, or support groups can provide motivation and accountability. Engaging with others who are on a similar journey fosters a sense of community and encourages individuals to remain committed to their weight loss goals. Regular check-ins with a partner or group can also help in reassessing strategies and making necessary adjustments to ensure continued progress.

By combining personal tracking methods with communal support, individuals can enhance their chances of achieving and maintaining permanent weight loss.

Chapter 3: Step Two - Sustainable Meal Planning

Creating Balanced Meal Plans

Creating balanced meal plans is a pivotal step in achieving and maintaining a healthy weight. For women navigating various life stages, such as pregnancy or menopause, and for busy professionals and new parents, understanding the components of a nutritious diet can make a significant difference in overall health and weight management. A balanced meal plan includes a variety of food groups that provide essential nutrients, which can help prevent cravings and promote satiety. By incorporating whole grains, lean proteins, healthy fats, and a colorful array of fruits and vegetables, individuals can optimize their meals for both health and weight loss.

When designing a meal plan, it is vital to consider caloric intake and nutritional density. Many health-conscious individuals overlook the importance of portion control, leading to unintentional overeating. Mindful eating techniques can be integrated into meal planning by encouraging individuals to focus on their hunger cues and eat slowly. This practice not only enhances the enjoyment of food but also aids in recognizing when one is satisfied. Balancing macronutrients—carbohydrates, proteins, and fats—in each meal can help stabilize blood sugar levels, reducing energy crashes and minimizing the temptation to snack on unhealthy options.

Flexibility is another crucial element in creating sustainable meal plans. Life can be unpredictable, and rigid diets often lead to frustration and disillusionment. By planning for a variety of meals and snacks, individuals can accommodate their schedules and cravings while still adhering to their health goals. Batch cooking or preparing meals in advance can save time during busy weeks, ensuring that nutritious options are readily available. Additionally, including a few indulgent meals in the plan can prevent feelings of deprivation, making it easier to stick to healthier choices overall.

The role of hydration should not be underestimated in the context of meal planning. Drinking enough water throughout the day is essential for metabolism and can aid in appetite regulation. Sometimes, feelings of hunger can be mistaken for thirst, leading to unnecessary snacking. Incorporating hydrating foods, such as fruits and vegetables, not only contributes to overall fluid intake but also provides essential vitamins and minerals that support health during various life stages. Encouraging individuals to make water their primary beverage can significantly impact their weight management efforts.

Lastly, building a support system can enhance the effectiveness of meal-planning strategies. Whether it's involving family members in the cooking process, sharing recipes with friends, or joining a community focused on health and wellness, having support can provide motivation and accountability. Engaging with others who share similar goals can lead to the exchange of ideas, encouragement during challenging moments, and a greater sense of achievement. By fostering a supportive environment, individuals can reinforce their commitment to balanced meal planning and ultimately achieve lasting weight loss success.

Incorporating Nutrient-Dense Foods

Incorporating nutrient-dense foods into your diet is a fundamental strategy for achieving permanent weight loss and maintaining overall health. These foods, rich in vitamins, minerals, and other beneficial compounds, provide the essential nutrients your body needs without the excess calories often found in processed options. For women navigating different life stages, such as menopause or pregnancy, nutrient-dense foods can help manage weight while addressing specific nutritional needs. By prioritizing these foods, you can enhance your energy levels, support metabolic functions, and promote sustained weight loss.

One effective approach to integrating nutrient-dense foods is to focus on whole, unprocessed ingredients. This includes fruits, vegetables, whole grains, lean proteins, and healthy fats. Planning meals around these foods can significantly improve the quality of your diet. For instance, starting your day with a smoothie made from leafy greens, berries, and a protein source can set a positive tone for your eating habits. Likewise, incorporating colorful vegetables into meals not only boosts nutrient intake but also adds variety and flavor, making healthy eating more enjoyable and sustainable.

Mindful eating techniques play a crucial role in ensuring that you fully appreciate and enjoy the nutrient-dense foods you include in your meals. Being present during meals allows you to listen to your body's hunger cues and recognize when you are satisfied. This practice can help prevent overeating and encourage a more positive relationship with food. By savoring each bite and acknowledging the flavors and textures of your meals, you can cultivate an appreciation for healthy foods and enhance your overall dietary experience.

For busy professionals and new parents, meal planning is an essential tool for incorporating nutrient-dense foods into daily routines. Preparing meals in advance allows you to have healthy options readily available, reducing the temptation to opt for convenient but less nutritious choices. Investing time in batch cooking and portioning out meals can simplify your week and ensure that you always have nourishing foods on hand. This proactive approach not only supports weight management but also fosters healthier eating habits for the entire family.

Finally, building a support system can significantly enhance your efforts to incorporate nutrient-dense foods into your lifestyle. Engaging with like-minded individuals, whether through fitness classes, community groups, or online platforms, can provide motivation and accountability. Sharing recipes, meal ideas, and progress with others can make the journey toward healthier eating more enjoyable and less isolating. By surrounding yourself with a supportive network, you increase your chances of long-term success in weight management and overall health.

Meal Prep Strategies for Busy Lifestyles

Meal prep can be a game changer for individuals juggling busy lifestyles, particularly for women managing weight during various life stages. The foundation of effective meal prep involves planning meals in advance, which not only saves time but also ensures that healthy options are readily available. Start by dedicating a specific day each week for meal planning and grocery shopping. This allows you to create a structured approach to your meals, reducing the likelihood of impulsive eating or resorting to unhealthy takeout options. By mapping out the week's meals, you can align your eating habits with your weight management goals.

Incorporating batch cooking into your meal prep strategy can significantly streamline your week. Prepare larger quantities of staple foods such as grains, proteins, and vegetables that can be easily mixed and matched throughout the week. For instance, cooking a big batch of quinoa, grilling several chicken breasts, and roasting a variety of vegetables can provide a versatile base for different meals. This approach not only minimizes cooking time but also allows for creative combinations, keeping meals exciting while remaining nutritious.

Utilizing storage containers effectively is another key strategy for successful meal prep. Invest in a variety of containers that are portion-controlled and microwave-safe, making it easy to reheat meals. Labeling containers with the date and meal type can help you keep track of freshness and ensure that you consume meals promptly. Additionally, consider preparing individual portions for snacks, like cut vegetables or homemade energy bites, to have healthy options on hand for busy days. This organization promotes mindful eating, as it reduces the temptation to grab high-calorie snacks in moments of hunger.

Incorporating seasonal produce into your meal prep can enhance both nutrition and flavor. Planning meals around what is in season not only supports local agriculture but also ensures that you are consuming fruits and vegetables at their peak freshness. This can be particularly beneficial for maintaining a balanced diet while managing weight. Explore farmers' markets or join a community-supported agriculture (CSA) program to access fresh, seasonal ingredients that can inspire your weekly meal plans.

Finally, adapting your meal prep strategy to accommodate your lifestyle changes is essential for long-term success. As life stages evolve, so too should your meal prep techniques. New parents might focus on quick, nutrient-dense options, while fitness enthusiasts may prioritize post-workout recovery meals. Regularly reassessing your meal prep approach ensures that it remains aligned with your goals, making it easier to sustain healthy eating habits over time. By integrating these meal prep strategies into your routine, you can create a sustainable framework for permanent weight loss that adapts to your busy lifestyle.

Chapter 4: Step Three - Mindful Eating Techniques

Understanding Hunger Cues

Understanding hunger cues is a fundamental aspect of achieving and maintaining a healthy weight. Hunger is not merely a physical sensation; it involves a complex interplay of physiological and psychological signals that can vary throughout different life stages. For women, factors such as hormonal fluctuations during menstruation, pregnancy, and menopause can significantly influence appetite and cravings. Recognizing these cues is essential for making informed dietary choices and fostering a healthier relationship with food.

The first step in understanding hunger cues is differentiating between true hunger and emotional eating. True hunger is characterized by physical symptoms such as a rumbling stomach, low energy levels, or difficulty concentrating. In contrast, emotional eating is often triggered by stress, boredom, or social situations. Identifying the root cause of your hunger can aid in developing mindful eating practices. By pausing to evaluate whether you are genuinely hungry or seeking comfort, you can make better choices that align with your long-term weight management goals.

Mindful eating techniques play a crucial role in interpreting hunger cues effectively. Slowing down during meals, savoring each bite, and tuning into your body's signals can enhance awareness of when you are satisfied. This practice not only helps prevent overeating but also encourages a deeper appreciation for the food you consume. Keeping a food journal can further assist in recognizing patterns in eating behaviors, including how different life circumstances affect your hunger levels and food choices.

For busy professionals and new parents, stress and time constraints can complicate the ability to heed hunger signals. It's common to overlook hunger cues when juggling multiple responsibilities, leading to binge eating or unhealthy snacking. Therefore, creating a structured eating schedule and prioritizing nutritious, easily accessible meals can help maintain balance. Incorporating quick, healthy snacks can also bridge the gap and ensure that you are not left overly hungry, which often leads to poor choices.

In conclusion, understanding hunger cues is vital for sustainable weight management across various life stages and circumstances. By learning to recognize the difference between physical hunger and emotional triggers, practicing mindful eating, and addressing the challenges posed by busy lifestyles, individuals can cultivate a healthier approach to food. This awareness not only supports weight loss efforts but also contributes to overall well-being and a more empowering relationship with food.

Eating with Intention

Eating with intention is a transformative approach to weight management that goes beyond merely counting calories or following strict diets. It involves a conscious effort to understand the reasons behind food choices, fostering a deeper connection to what we consume. For women navigating different life stages, such as menopause or pregnancy, this approach can be particularly beneficial. It allows for a greater awareness of how hormonal changes can affect cravings and energy levels, enabling individuals to make informed decisions that support their unique health needs.

Mindful eating techniques are at the core of eating with intention. This practice encourages individuals to slow down during meals, paying attention to the flavors, textures, and aromas of food. By focusing on each bite, you can cultivate a heightened awareness of hunger and fullness cues, which is essential for preventing overeating. For busy professionals and new parents, carving out time for meals can be challenging, but setting aside just a few moments to breathe and appreciate your food can create a more satisfying eating experience, ultimately aiding in weight loss efforts.

Sustainable meal planning is another critical aspect of intentional eating. By preparing balanced meals in advance, you can avoid the pitfalls of last-minute, often unhealthy food choices. This becomes particularly important for fitness enthusiasts and those managing health conditions who require specific nutrients. Incorporating a variety of whole foods—such as fruits, vegetables, lean proteins, and whole grains—into your meal plans not only supports weight loss but also helps in maintaining energy levels throughout the day.

Emotional eating is a common hurdle for many individuals on their weight loss journey. Recognizing triggers, whether they stem from stress, boredom, or other emotions, is vital for overcoming this challenge. Strategies from experts suggest developing alternative coping mechanisms, such as engaging in physical activity or practicing relaxation techniques. By identifying and addressing emotional eating patterns, you can cultivate a more intentional relationship with food, ensuring that meals are driven by physical hunger rather than emotional needs.

Lastly, integrating fitness and nutrition plays a significant role in achieving lasting weight loss. Eating with intention complements an active lifestyle, allowing individuals—regardless of their fitness levels—to fuel their bodies appropriately. Understanding how different foods affect performance and recovery can enhance workout results, making it easier to stick with a routine. Building a support system, whether through friends, family, or online communities, can further reinforce these habits, creating a sustainable framework for long-term weight management.

Techniques for Practicing Mindfulness

Techniques for practicing mindfulness can significantly enhance your weight management journey by fostering a deeper connection between your mind and body. Mindfulness encourages individuals to focus on the present moment, which is essential when making decisions about food and exercise. By incorporating mindfulness into your daily routine, you can improve your awareness of hunger cues, emotional triggers, and overall physical sensations, all of which play a critical role in sustainable weight loss.

One effective technique is mindful eating, where you slow down and pay attention to the sensory experience of food. This involves engaging all your senses while eating—taking note of the colors, textures, and aromas of your meals. Eating without distractions, such as television or smartphones, allows you to fully appreciate what you consume. By doing so, you are more likely to recognize when you are satisfied, which can prevent overeating and promote healthier food choices.

Another vital mindfulness practice is meditation, which can help reduce stress and anxiety, both of which can lead to emotional eating. Setting aside just a few minutes each day to meditate can clear your mind and help you cultivate a sense of calm. Guided meditations focused on weight loss or body positivity can be particularly beneficial. As you develop this practice, you may find it easier to approach food choices with a more balanced mindset, rather than being driven by stress or negative emotions.

Incorporating mindfulness into your physical activity is also essential. Whether you are engaging in a home workout or a walk in the park, focus on how your body feels during the exercise. Pay attention to your breath, the rhythm of your movements, and the sensations in your muscles. This heightened awareness can make your workouts more enjoyable and effective, as you learn to listen to your body and adjust your routine based on its needs.

Lastly, journaling can serve as a powerful mindfulness technique. Writing down your thoughts, feelings, and experiences related to food and exercise can provide insights into your behaviors and patterns. Reflecting on your emotions can help you identify triggers for emotional eating and facilitate a more mindful approach to your diet and fitness regimen. By documenting your journey, you can track your progress and cultivate a greater sense of accountability, ultimately leading to lasting weight management success.

Chapter 5: Step Four - Home Workouts for Weight Management

Designing an Effective Home Workout Routine

Designing an effective home workout routine requires a thoughtful approach that considers individual fitness levels, lifestyle constraints, and specific weight management goals. The foundation of any successful routine begins with understanding personal capabilities and preferences. Women, in particular, may experience varying energy levels and physical limitations during different life stages, such as pregnancy or menopause.

By recognizing these factors, individuals can tailor their workouts to include a mix of cardiovascular exercises, strength training, and flexibility work that suits their unique situations.

Incorporating a variety of exercises can prevent boredom and enhance overall effectiveness. For busy professionals and new parents, time-efficient workouts that can be completed in 30 minutes or less can be particularly appealing. High-Intensity Interval Training (HIIT) can be an excellent option, as it allows for maximum calorie burn in a short period. Additionally, integrating bodyweight exercises such as squats, lunges, and push-ups can be effective without the need for expensive equipment. Fitness enthusiasts and those who engage in regular activity can benefit from progressive overload, gradually increasing the intensity or duration of workouts to continue seeing results.

Setting realistic and achievable goals is essential for maintaining motivation and tracking progress. Whether aiming to lose a specific number of pounds, improve endurance, or build strength, clearly defined objectives provide direction. For individuals with health conditions or seniors, it's crucial to consult with healthcare professionals before starting any new routine. This ensures that the chosen exercises are safe and beneficial, allowing for adjustments that cater to specific health concerns while still promoting weight loss and fitness.

Mindful eating should complement the workout routine to create a holistic approach to weight management. Being aware of nutritional choices can enhance the benefits of exercise, helping individuals fuel their bodies properly for workouts and recovery. For those working on overcoming emotional eating, combining workout sessions with mindfulness techniques can foster a positive relationship with food and exercise. Establishing a consistent schedule that integrates both physical activity and healthy eating habits can lead to sustainable weight loss and long-term success.

Finally, building a support system can significantly enhance the journey toward achieving weight management goals. Connecting with friends, family, or online communities can provide encouragement and accountability. Sharing successes and challenges can motivate individuals to stay on track and reinvigorate their commitment to their fitness routines. In summary, designing an effective home workout routine involves understanding personal needs, incorporating diverse exercises, setting achievable goals, practicing mindful eating, and fostering a supportive environment to ensure lasting weight loss success.

Utilizing Bodyweight Exercises

Utilizing bodyweight exercises is a highly effective strategy for women and men alike looking to manage their weight while adapting to various life stages and circumstances. These exercises leverage one's body weight for resistance, eliminating the need for costly gym memberships or elaborate equipment.

Whether you are navigating the challenges of pregnancy, experiencing the changes of menopause, or simply juggling a busy lifestyle, bodyweight exercises offer scalable options that can fit seamlessly into your daily routine.

They can be performed anywhere, making it easier to incorporate physical activity into your life without the barriers that often accompany traditional workouts.

One of the key benefits of bodyweight exercises is their versatility. They can be modified to suit different fitness levels, from beginners to advanced practitioners. For busy professionals or new parents, short, high-intensity bodyweight workouts can deliver significant results in a fraction of the time compared to traditional methods. Exercises such as squats, push-ups, and lunges can be adjusted in difficulty, allowing individuals to progressively challenge themselves as they build strength and endurance. This adaptability makes bodyweight training an excellent option for those who may have specific health conditions or physical limitations, providing a pathway to fitness that is both safe and effective.

In addition to physical benefits, bodyweight exercises can also enhance mental well-being. Engaging in regular physical activity has been shown to release endorphins, which can help combat stress and improve mood. For individuals facing emotional eating challenges or the psychological impacts of weight management, incorporating bodyweight exercises into a routine can serve as a constructive outlet. The satisfaction of accomplishing a workout can foster a sense of achievement and motivation, reinforcing a positive relationship with fitness and nutrition.

Another significant advantage of bodyweight exercises is their role in building functional strength. As women and men progress through different life stages, maintaining strength and mobility becomes increasingly important. Bodyweight training emphasizes functional movements that mimic everyday activities, which can help improve balance, coordination, and overall physical performance. This is particularly crucial for seniors who may be looking to maintain independence and for young adults who seek a solid foundation for athletic pursuits. By focusing on movements that translate to real-life scenarios, bodyweight exercises can contribute to long-term health and well-being.

To integrate bodyweight exercises effectively into a weight management plan, consistency is key. Establishing a regular workout schedule that includes these exercises alongside mindful eating and sustainable nutrition practices can create a comprehensive approach to weight loss. Setting achievable goals and tracking progress can motivate while fostering accountability. As you embrace bodyweight workouts, remember that the journey to permanent weight loss is not just about the numbers on the scale; it's about cultivating a healthier lifestyle that supports your unique needs and aspirations.

Incorporating Flexibility and Strength Training

Incorporating flexibility and strength training into a fitness regimen is crucial for effective weight management, particularly for women navigating various life stages. Flexibility exercises, such as yoga or dynamic stretching, enhance the range of motion in joints and muscles. This is particularly important during periods like menopause, where hormonal changes can lead to stiffness and decreased mobility. By integrating flexibility training into their routine, women can not only alleviate discomfort but also improve their overall performance in strength training and cardiovascular activities, ultimately supporting their weight loss goals.

Strength training is equally vital in a comprehensive weight management strategy. It helps build lean muscle mass, which is essential for boosting metabolism. Women, especially as they age, may experience muscle loss, leading to a slower metabolic rate. By incorporating resistance exercises such as weight lifting, bodyweight workouts, or resistance bands, individuals can combat this decline.

This shift not only aids in calorie burning during workouts but also continues to elevate metabolism for hours post-exercise, contributing to more effective weight loss and maintenance.

For busy professionals and new parents, finding time for both flexibility and strength training can seem daunting. However, these exercises can easily be integrated into daily routines. Short, high-intensity strength workouts can be completed in 20-30 minutes, and flexibility exercises can be performed at home during short breaks or even while watching television. This adaptability ensures that even the busiest individuals can prioritize their fitness without feeling overwhelmed, making sustainable weight loss more achievable.

Mindful eating practices can also complement a fitness regimen focused on flexibility and strength. Being aware of one's body and its needs encourages individuals to listen to hunger cues and choose nutritious foods that support their training efforts. This awareness can help prevent emotional eating, a common challenge for many. When women align their fitness goals with mindful eating, they create a holistic approach to weight management that is both practical and effective.

Finally, it's essential to build a support system that encourages consistency in both flexibility and strength training. Engaging with fitness communities, whether online or in person, can provide motivation and accountability. Sharing progress, challenges, and successes can foster a sense of camaraderie and commitment. By cultivating an environment that values both physical fitness and nutrition, women can enhance their chances of achieving permanent weight loss, making these practices not just a temporary solution but a lasting lifestyle change.

Chapter 6: Step Five - Overcoming Emotional Eating

Identifying Triggers for Emotional Eating

Identifying the triggers for emotional eating is a crucial step in managing weight effectively. Emotional eating often stems from various feelings, including stress, anxiety, loneliness, or even boredom. For many individuals, food becomes a source of comfort during challenging times, leading to patterns that can undermine weight loss efforts. Recognizing these emotional triggers is essential for developing strategies to combat them. By understanding the underlying emotions that prompt the urge to eat, individuals can begin to address the root causes rather than simply reacting with food.

One common trigger for emotional eating is stress. Many women, particularly those navigating life transitions such as pregnancy or menopause, may find themselves dealing with heightened stress levels. As responsibilities increase and hormonal changes occur, food can become a quick escape from overwhelming feelings. Identifying specific stressors, whether they are related to work, family, or personal expectations, allows individuals to create healthier coping mechanisms. This might involve engaging in physical activity, practicing mindfulness, or seeking social support rather than turning to food for relief.

Another significant trigger is emotional fatigue or boredom. In today's fast-paced world, busy professionals and new parents often experience exhaustion that can lead to mindless eating. Recognizing the difference between true hunger and emotional fatigue is vital. Keeping a food diary can help individuals track when and why they eat, providing insights into patterns of emotional eating. By becoming more aware of these behaviors, individuals can implement strategies such as planned snacking or engaging in alternative activities that provide fulfillment without resorting to food.

Social situations can also trigger emotional eating. Meals and gatherings often become venues for indulging in comfort foods, and the pressure to conform to social norms can lead to overeating. Understanding the dynamics of social eating is important for maintaining weight loss goals. Developing assertiveness around food choices and learning to enjoy social interactions without relying on food can significantly impact one's relationship with eating. Strategies such as bringing healthy dishes to gatherings or practicing mindful eating during meals can help maintain focus on nutritional choices.

Lastly, hormonal fluctuations during different life stages can contribute to emotional eating. For instance, women may experience cravings linked to hormonal changes during their menstrual cycles or menopause. Recognizing these patterns can empower individuals to prepare for these fluctuations by having healthy snacks on hand or planning meals that stabilize mood and energy levels. By identifying these hormonal triggers and understanding their impact on emotional eating, individuals can develop a more proactive approach to managing their weight and promoting overall well-being.

Strategies to Manage Emotional Eating

Emotional eating can be a significant barrier to achieving and maintaining weight loss goals, especially for women navigating various life stages such as menopause, pregnancy, or the challenges of motherhood. To effectively manage emotional eating, it is essential to first recognize the triggers that lead to this behavior. Common triggers include stress, boredom, fatigue, or even emotional distress. Keeping a food diary can be a valuable tool in identifying patterns associated with emotional eating. By tracking what you eat, when you eat, and how you feel during those moments, you can gain insights into the emotional connections tied to your eating habits.

Once triggers are identified, developing alternative coping strategies is crucial. Instead of turning to food for comfort, consider engaging in activities that provide emotional relief. This could involve physical exercise, which not only boosts endorphins but also serves as a productive outlet for stress. Other options might include practicing mindfulness techniques such as meditation or deep breathing exercises.

These practices can help you reconnect with your emotions and manage them without resorting to food. Additionally, hobbies such as reading, painting, or gardening can serve as fulfilling distractions that keep you engaged and away from the refrigerator.

Another effective strategy is to build a supportive environment that promotes healthy eating habits. Surrounding yourself with friends or family members who understand your goals can provide emotional support and accountability. Consider joining a local weight loss group or online community where members share similar challenges and successes. This network can offer motivation and encouragement, making it easier to resist the urge to eat emotionally. H

aving a buddy system in place can also help in making healthier choices together, whether it's planning meals or engaging in physical activities.

Mindful eating is a powerful technique to combat emotional eating. This practice encourages individuals to pay attention to their eating experience, focusing on the taste, texture, and aroma of food. By slowing down and savoring each bite, you become more aware of your body's hunger and fullness cues. This heightened awareness can help differentiate between physical hunger and emotional cravings. Implementing mindful eating can create a more satisfying relationship with food, where every meal is an opportunity to enjoy and appreciate nourishment rather than a means to fill emotional voids.

Lastly, addressing the role of sleep in emotional eating cannot be overlooked. Lack of adequate sleep can lead to increased stress levels and poor decision-making regarding food choices. Establishing a regular sleep schedule and creating a restful sleep environment can improve overall mood and reduce the likelihood of turning to food for comfort. Prioritizing sleep as a part of your weight management strategy not only supports physical health but also enhances emotional resilience, making it easier to navigate the ups and downs of life without relying on food as a coping mechanism.

Seeking Professional Help When Needed

Seeking professional help when managing weight can be a pivotal decision for individuals at various life stages. Whether you are navigating the changes of menopause, coping with the demands of new parenthood, or simply looking to shed pounds for a healthier lifestyle, guidance from experts can provide the necessary support and knowledge. Professionals such as registered dietitians, nutritionists, and personal trainers can offer tailored advice that aligns with individual health needs, preferences, and goals. Their expertise can help demystify the complexities of nutrition and exercise, making it easier to adopt sustainable practices.

Incorporating professional assistance can also be particularly beneficial during times of significant life changes. For instance, pregnant women and new mothers often face unique challenges related to weight management. A qualified nutritionist can help create meal plans that nourish both mother and baby while promoting healthy weight gain or loss.

Similarly, seniors may require specialized fitness programs that accommodate their physical capabilities and health conditions. Professionals can design individualized exercise regimens that not only support weight loss but also enhance overall mobility and strength.

Emotional eating is another area where professional help can make a significant difference. Many individuals turn to food as a coping mechanism during stressful times, leading to unhealthy eating patterns. Therapists and counselors trained in nutritional psychology can provide strategies to overcome these habits.

They can help clients identify triggers, develop mindful eating techniques, and build healthier relationships with food. Seeking this kind of support can lead to profound changes in behavior and mindset, paving the way for lasting weight loss success.

Support systems play a crucial role in weight management, and professionals can help establish these networks. Joining a weight loss program led by a trained expert can foster accountability and encouragement. Group settings often allow for shared experiences and collective motivation, which can be particularly empowering. Additionally, professionals can assist in building a personal support system, connecting individuals with others who share similar goals and challenges. This community aspect can enhance commitment to a weight loss journey and reinforce positive lifestyle changes.

In conclusion, reaching out for professional help is a proactive step toward achieving and maintaining weight loss goals. The guidance from experts can not only provide personalized advice but also instill confidence in one's abilities to navigate the complexities of weight management. By leveraging professional knowledge and support, individuals can embark on their weight loss journeys with a solid foundation, ensuring that their efforts lead to sustainable and lasting results.

Chapter 7: Integrating Fitness and Nutrition

The Synergy Between Diet and Exercise

The synergy between diet and exercise plays a critical role in achieving and maintaining permanent weight loss. Understanding how these two components interact can significantly enhance your approach to health and fitness, particularly for women navigating different life stages such as menopause or pregnancy. A balanced diet provides the necessary nutrients and energy required for effective workout sessions, while regular physical activity boosts metabolism and aids in calorie expenditure.

When these elements are harmoniously integrated, they create a powerful framework for sustainable weight management.

Effective meal planning is essential for supporting an active lifestyle. Busy professionals and new parents often struggle to find the time for both exercise and proper nutrition. By preparing meals in advance and focusing on nutrient-dense foods, individuals can ensure they have the fuel needed to power through workouts. Lean proteins, whole grains, fruits, and vegetables should form the foundation of a balanced diet. This not only enhances energy levels but also helps to regulate hunger and prevent unhealthy snacking, making it easier to stay on track with weight loss goals.

Incorporating mindful eating techniques can further amplify the effects of exercise on weight loss. By paying attention to hunger cues and savoring each bite, individuals can foster a healthier relationship with food. This practice helps combat emotional eating, a common challenge for many, including busy professionals and new parents. When combined with regular physical activity, mindful eating contributes to a more intentional approach to weight management, aiding in the development of sustainable habits that last over time.

The role of sleep in this synergy cannot be overlooked. Quality sleep is vital for recovery, hormone regulation, and overall well-being. Poor sleep can lead to increased cravings and reduced motivation to exercise, creating a cycle that can hinder weight loss efforts. For those striving for lasting results, prioritizing sleep alongside a balanced diet and regular workouts is crucial. Establishing a routine that includes adequate rest will enhance energy levels, improve exercise performance, and support the body's recovery processes.

Building a support system is also key to navigating the complexities of weight loss, particularly for women experiencing hormonal changes or those managing health conditions. Engaging with like-minded individuals can provide accountability and encouragement. Whether through group workouts, online forums, or community classes, sharing experiences and strategies can foster a sense of belonging. This collaborative environment not only motivates individuals to stay committed to their diet and exercise regimes but also reinforces the understanding that achieving weight loss success is a multifaceted journey requiring both effort and support.

Customizing Your Fitness Regimen

Customizing your fitness regimen is essential for achieving sustainable weight loss and overall well-being. The first step in tailoring your fitness plan is to assess your current lifestyle, goals, and any unique circumstances you may face. For example, women experiencing menopause may need to incorporate strength training to counteract muscle loss, while busy professionals might benefit from high-intensity interval training (HIIT) that maximizes efficiency in a limited timeframe. Understanding your starting point allows you to create a regimen that is both enjoyable and effective, making it easier to stick with in the long term.

Next, consider integrating a mix of cardiovascular, strength, and flexibility exercises into your routine. Cardiovascular workouts such as walking, running, or cycling can help burn calories and improve heart health, while strength training builds muscle and boosts metabolism. Flexibility exercises, like yoga or stretching, not only enhance physical performance but also promote relaxation and stress relief, which are critical for emotional well-being. By balancing these components, you create a comprehensive fitness regimen that addresses multiple aspects of health and weight management.

Another crucial factor in customizing your fitness regimen is setting realistic and achievable goals. Aim for specific, measurable outcomes rather than vague aspirations. For instance, instead of simply wishing to "get fit," set a goal to run a 5K in three months or to complete a specific number of strength training sessions each week. Break these larger goals into smaller milestones to track progress and celebrate achievements along the way. This practice fosters motivation and helps maintain focus, especially during challenging times.

Incorporating mindfulness into your fitness routine can also enhance the customization process. Mindful movement encourages you to be present during workouts, allowing you to listen to your body and adjust exercises based on how you feel. This approach helps prevent injuries and ensures you are working within your limits, particularly important for those with health conditions or new parents who may have fluctuating energy levels. Mindful practices can also extend to your nutrition, helping you develop a holistic approach to weight management.

Lastly, establishing a support system can significantly impact the success of your customized fitness regimen. Connect with friends, family, or online communities that share similar goals and challenges. This network can provide encouragement, accountability, and advice tailored to your unique situation. Participating in group classes or finding a workout buddy can also make exercising more enjoyable and less isolating. Remember, the journey to permanent weight loss is not just about physical changes but also about building a sustainable lifestyle that supports your long-term health and well-being.

Nutritional Timing and Its Impact

Nutritional timing refers to the strategic planning of meals and snacks throughout the day to optimize body function and enhance weight management. This concept is particularly relevant for women navigating various life stages, as hormonal fluctuations can significantly influence metabolism, hunger signals, and energy levels. By understanding when to eat and what to consume, women can better manage their weight and overall health.

For instance, during menopause, the body's metabolism may slow down, making it essential to adjust meal timing to prevent unwanted weight gain. Eating larger meals earlier in the day when energy expenditure is typically higher can be an effective strategy.

For busy professionals and new parents, time constraints often lead to irregular eating patterns, which can disrupt metabolism and promote weight gain. Implementing a structured meal schedule can help mitigate these issues. Planning meals around work schedules or family obligations ensures that nutritious options are available when hunger strikes. Additionally, incorporating healthy snacks between meals can prevent overeating at mealtimes and help maintain stable blood sugar levels, which is crucial for sustained energy and appetite control.

Athletes and fitness enthusiasts can leverage nutritional timing to enhance performance and recovery. Consuming a balanced meal or snack rich in carbohydrates and protein before and after workouts can support energy levels and muscle repair. This is particularly important for those engaged in intense training or competitive sports, as optimal nutrient intake can lead to improved performance outcomes.

By timing nutrient consumption around exercise, individuals can maximize their physical potential while also promoting effective weight management.

Mindful eating techniques are also essential when considering nutritional timing. Being aware of hunger cues and ensuring that meals are consumed without distractions can lead to greater satisfaction and reduced calorie intake. Engaging in the practice of mindful eating allows individuals to better recognize the appropriate times to eat and when to stop, fostering a healthier relationship with food. This is especially beneficial for those dealing with emotional eating or stress-related food choices, as it encourages a focus on the body's true nutritional needs.

In conclusion, nutritional timing plays a crucial role in effective weight management for diverse populations. By understanding the timing of meals and snacks, individuals can tailor their eating habits to their unique lifestyle needs, ensuring they remain satisfied and energized throughout the day. Whether it's coordinating meals around a busy work schedule, enhancing athletic performance, or managing hormonal changes, strategic nutritional timing can serve as a powerful tool in the journey toward sustainable weight loss.

Chapter 8: The Role of Sleep in Weight Loss

Understanding Sleep's Impact on Metabolism

Sleep plays a crucial role in regulating metabolism, which significantly influences weight management. During sleep, the body undergoes various restorative processes that affect hormonal balance and energy expenditure. When sleep is compromised, whether due to stress, lifestyle choices, or health conditions, it can lead to hormonal imbalances, particularly with hormones like leptin and ghrelin. Leptin, which signals satiety, decreases with inadequate sleep, while ghrelin, responsible for hunger, increases.

This shift can lead to increased appetite and cravings, making it challenging to maintain a healthy diet and weight.

Moreover, insufficient sleep can affect insulin sensitivity, which is vital for glucose metabolism. When the body is deprived of sleep, it may become less effective at processing glucose, leading to higher blood sugar levels. This can contribute to weight gain and increase the risk of metabolic disorders, such as type 2 diabetes. For busy professionals and new parents, who often experience irregular sleep patterns, understanding this relationship is essential in developing strategies to improve both sleep quality and metabolic health.

The impact of sleep on metabolism extends to energy levels and motivation. A well-rested individual is more likely to engage in physical activity, whereas sleep deprivation can lead to fatigue and decreased motivation to exercise. For fitness enthusiasts and athletes, this can hinder performance and recovery, making it critical to prioritize sleep as part of a comprehensive fitness regimen. Incorporating restorative sleep practices can enhance workout efficiency and overall energy balance, supporting long-term weight loss goals.

Additionally, sleep quality is linked to emotional well-being, which can affect food choices and eating behaviors. When individuals are tired, they may resort to unhealthy snacks for quick energy boosts or comfort foods to cope with stress. This pattern can create a cycle of emotional eating that complicates weight management efforts. By focusing on improving sleep hygiene and establishing consistent sleep routines, individuals can foster better emotional health and make more mindful eating decisions.

In conclusion, understanding the intricate relationship between sleep and metabolism is vital for anyone looking to manage their weight effectively. By prioritizing sleep as a foundational aspect of a healthy lifestyle, individuals can enhance their metabolic function, improve hormonal balance, and support their overall weight loss and maintenance efforts. Emphasizing sleep alongside nutrition and exercise creates a holistic approach to achieving lasting results in weight management.

Establishing Healthy Sleep Habits

Establishing healthy sleep habits is a crucial yet often overlooked component of effective weight management. Sleep plays a significant role in regulating hormones that control appetite, metabolism, and energy levels. Insufficient sleep can lead to an increase in ghrelin, the hunger hormone while decreasing leptin, which signals fullness. This hormonal imbalance often results in cravings for high-calorie foods and can derail even the most dedicated weight-loss efforts. By prioritizing quality sleep, individuals can create a solid foundation for achieving and maintaining their weight loss goals.

Creating an optimal sleep environment is the first step toward better sleep hygiene. This involves minimizing distractions and creating a calm atmosphere conducive to rest. Consider factors such as room temperature, lighting, and noise levels. A cool, dark, and quiet room can significantly enhance sleep quality. Additionally, investing in a comfortable mattress and pillows tailored to personal preferences can improve comfort levels. Establishing a regular bedtime routine can signal to the body that it's time to wind down, making it easier to fall asleep and stay asleep.

Screen time before bed can severely impact sleep quality. The blue light emitted by phones, tablets, and computers can interfere with the production of melatonin, the hormone responsible for regulating sleep-wake cycles. To combat this, it's advisable to set boundaries around technology use, particularly in the hour leading up to bedtime. Instead, consider engaging in calming activities such as reading, meditating, or practicing gentle yoga. These activities can help to reduce stress and prepare both the mind and body for restorative sleep.

Mindful eating practices can also be connected to sleep health. Eating too close to bedtime can disrupt sleep patterns, especially if the meal is heavy or high in sugar. Establishing a routine that includes a consistent last meal of the day can help regulate both appetite and sleep. Aim to finish eating at least two to three hours before bedtime, allowing the body ample time to digest food. This not only promotes better sleep but also aids in metabolic processes that are essential for weight loss.

Finally, understanding the connection between sleep and physical activity can further enhance weight management efforts. Regular exercise promotes better sleep quality and can help regulate appetite. However, timing is essential; engaging in vigorous workouts too close to bedtime may lead to difficulty falling asleep. Finding the right balance between physical activity and rest is key. By integrating healthy sleep habits into daily routines, individuals can create a supportive environment for weight loss, ultimately leading to a healthier lifestyle that is sustainable over the long term.

Addressing Sleep Disorders

Sleep disorders can significantly impact weight management efforts, making it essential to address these issues to achieve lasting results. Quality sleep is vital for regulating hormones that control appetite, such as ghrelin and leptin. When sleep is compromised, ghrelin levels can rise, increasing hunger, while leptin levels fall, reducing the feeling of fullness. This hormonal imbalance can lead to overeating, poor food choices, and ultimately, weight gain. Therefore, understanding how to improve sleep quality can be a critical step in the journey toward permanent weight loss.

Identifying common sleep disorders is the first step in addressing these issues. Conditions such as insomnia, sleep apnea, and restless leg syndrome can disrupt sleep patterns and affect overall health. For women, hormonal fluctuations during menopause can exacerbate sleep disturbances, making it even more crucial to find effective solutions. By paying attention to sleep patterns and seeking professional help when necessary, individuals can begin to tackle these disorders head-on, setting the stage for more effective weight management.

Incorporating healthy sleep habits into daily routines can also play a significant role in promoting better sleep quality. Establishing a consistent sleep schedule, creating a relaxing bedtime routine, and designing a sleep-friendly environment can help signal to the body that it's time to wind down. Limiting screen time before bed, avoiding caffeine in the afternoon, and engaging in relaxation techniques such as meditation or deep breathing can further enhance sleep quality. These adjustments not only improve sleep but also support overall health, making it easier to maintain a healthy weight.

Nutrition and sleep are closely linked, and making mindful dietary choices can positively impact sleep quality. Consuming a balanced diet rich in whole foods, including fruits, vegetables, whole grains, and lean proteins, can promote better sleep patterns. Additionally, certain foods, such as almonds, turkey, and chamomile tea, contain sleep-promoting compounds that can help individuals fall asleep faster and stay asleep longer. By integrating these foods into meal planning, individuals can support both their sleep and weight loss goals simultaneously.

Finally, building a support system that includes discussions about sleep can provide additional motivation and accountability. Sharing experiences and strategies with friends, family, or support groups can help individuals stay committed to improving their sleep habits. By recognizing the integral role sleep plays in weight management, individuals can approach their weight loss journey holistically, ensuring they address all aspects of their health for sustainable results.

Chapter 9: Building a Support System

The Importance of Community in Weight Loss

Community plays a critical role in the journey of weight loss, influencing motivation, accountability, and emotional support. For women navigating various life stages such as menopause or pregnancy, having a supportive network can make a significant difference in their ability to manage weight effectively. The shared experiences and challenges faced by individuals in similar situations foster a sense of belonging and understanding. This connection can alleviate feelings of isolation that often accompany weight loss efforts, encouraging individuals to persist in their goals.

One of the primary benefits of community in weight loss is the accountability it provides. When individuals engage with others who share similar health and fitness aspirations, they are more likely to stay committed to their plans. Group challenges, whether in-person or online, create a sense of urgency and collective motivation.

For busy professionals or new parents, scheduling regular check-ins or group workouts can help maintain focus and consistency in their routines, making weight management more achievable amid their hectic lives.

Moreover, communities can serve as valuable sources of information and inspiration. Participants often share tips, recipes, and strategies that have worked for them, enriching the collective knowledge. For those interested in sustainable meal planning or mindful eating techniques, a community can provide practical advice and encouragement. Engaging with others can also introduce individuals to new workout ideas or nutrition plans that align with their personal goals, enhancing their overall weight loss journey.

Emotional eating is a challenge many face during weight loss, and community support can be instrumental in overcoming this hurdle. By connecting with others who understand the struggle, individuals can share their experiences and coping strategies. Support groups or forums can offer a safe space to discuss feelings and triggers, making it easier to develop healthier relationships with food.

This mutual support can empower individuals to recognize their emotional eating patterns and work collaboratively toward healthier behaviors.

Lastly, building a community is not just about social support; it can also create a positive environment that promotes long-term lifestyle changes. Whether through organized fitness classes, online forums, or informal meet-ups, the sense of camaraderie can transform the weight loss experience from a solitary endeavor into a shared journey.

As individuals celebrate each other's successes and provide encouragement during setbacks, they cultivate resilience and determination that are essential for achieving and maintaining weight loss goals over time.

Such a supportive network not only fuels motivation but also reinforces the idea that weight loss is a holistic process that thrives in a community-focused atmosphere.

Finding Accountability Partners

Finding the right accountability partner is a crucial component of any successful weight management journey. These individuals can provide support, encouragement, and motivation, helping you stay committed to your goals. Whether you're navigating the challenges of pregnancy, managing weight during menopause, or simply striving for a healthier lifestyle, having someone by your side can make a significant difference. An accountability partner can be a friend, family member, or even a colleague who shares similar health objectives, creating a mutually beneficial relationship where both parties can thrive.

When selecting an accountability partner, consider someone who understands your specific goals and the unique challenges you face. For busy professionals, this might mean finding another individual who also juggles work and family responsibilities. For fitness enthusiasts, it could be a workout buddy who shares your passion for exercise. It's important that your partner not only supports you but also inspires you to push beyond your limits. Look for someone who is positive, reliable, and committed, as these traits will help foster an environment of trust and encouragement.

Communication is key in any accountability partnership. Establish a regular check-in schedule, whether through phone calls, texts, or in-person meetings, to discuss progress, setbacks, and strategies for improvement. Use these conversations to celebrate achievements, no matter how small, and to brainstorm solutions for challenges that may arise. Open and honest communication can help you both stay focused and engaged in your weight loss journey, creating a sense of camaraderie that can be invaluable during tough times.

Incorporating shared activities can strengthen your partnership even further. Consider planning workouts together, cooking healthy meals, or attending fitness classes as a duo. Engaging in these activities not only makes the process more enjoyable but also reinforces your commitment to one another. Additionally, sharing resources such as meal planning ideas, recipes, or workout routines can provide both of you with fresh perspectives and strategies that may enhance your journeys toward sustainable weight loss.

Lastly, remember that accountability is a two-way street. While you may lean on your partner for motivation and support, be sure to reciprocate the same energy and encouragement. Celebrate their victories and provide a listening ear during challenging moments. This mutual support fosters a sense of community and can significantly enhance the likelihood of achieving your weight management goals. Embracing the journey together not only makes the process more enjoyable but also reinforces the commitment to lasting change, ultimately leading to successful outcomes for both partners.

Utilizing Online Resources and Groups

Utilizing online resources and groups can significantly enhance your weight management journey, offering support, information, and a sense of community. The digital landscape is filled with forums, social media platforms, and websites dedicated to health and wellness, where individuals can find valuable tips, share their experiences, and connect with others facing similar challenges.

These platforms often feature discussions on topics such as sustainable meal planning and mindful eating techniques, allowing participants to gain insights that are especially relevant to their unique situations, whether they are navigating menopause, pregnancy, or other life stages.

Online communities not only provide information but also foster accountability and motivation. Many individuals find that sharing their goals and progress with a supportive group can be a powerful motivator. For instance, fitness enthusiasts may join groups focused on home workouts or weight loss challenges, discovering new routines and encouragement from peers.

Similarly, new parents can find solace in connecting with others who understand the demands of parenting while trying to maintain a healthy lifestyle. This supportive environment can be crucial in overcoming emotional eating and maintaining consistent progress.

Social media platforms such as Instagram and Facebook host numerous pages and groups dedicated to health and wellness. These spaces often share tips on integrating fitness and nutrition, debunking common weight loss myths, and offering advanced metabolism-boosting techniques. Engaging with content from professionals and knowledgeable peers can deepen your understanding of effective strategies for weight loss and healthy living. By following credible sources, you can stay informed about the latest research and trends, ensuring your approach is both effective and sustainable.

In addition to social media, there are various websites and apps designed to assist with meal planning and tracking progress. These resources often include features such as calorie counters, recipe databases, and workout logs. For busy professionals and health-conscious individuals, such tools can simplify the process of maintaining a balanced diet and regular exercise routine. Furthermore, some platforms provide personalized plans tailored to individual goals, making it easier to navigate dietary needs, especially for those with health conditions or specific fitness objectives.

Finally, participating in online groups can help build a support system that is vital for lasting weight loss success. Engaging with others who share similar experiences can lead to the exchange of practical strategies and emotional support. Whether it's celebrating small victories or finding encouragement during setbacks, the relationships formed in these communities can provide the strength needed to persevere. By utilizing these online resources effectively, individuals can create a well-rounded approach to weight management that encompasses education, motivation, and camaraderie, ultimately leading to lasting results.

Chapter 10: Advanced Metabolism Boosting Techniques

Understanding Metabolism and Its Factors

Metabolism refers to the complex biochemical processes through which the body converts food into energy. Understanding metabolism is crucial for anyone looking to manage weight effectively, as it directly influences how efficiently our bodies burn calories and utilize nutrients. Metabolism encompasses two primary components: catabolism, which breaks down food to release energy, and anabolism, which builds and stores essential compounds.

The balance between these processes is affected by various factors, including age, gender, body composition, hormonal levels, and lifestyle choices.

One of the most significant influences on metabolism is age. As individuals progress through different life stages, particularly women during menopause, metabolic rates tend to decline. This reduction can be attributed to hormonal changes that occur during menopause, leading to increased fat storage and decreased muscle mass. Consequently, understanding how metabolism shifts with age can empower individuals to adjust their dietary and exercise habits accordingly, promoting a more effective weight management strategy during transitional periods.

Body composition also plays a critical role in metabolic rate. Muscle tissue burns more calories at rest compared to fat tissue, which means that those with a higher muscle-to-fat ratio typically have a higher resting metabolic rate. Engaging in strength training can be particularly beneficial for increasing muscle mass and, in turn, boosting metabolism. Busy professionals and new parents may find it challenging to fit in workouts; however, incorporating resistance exercises into short, manageable routines can lead to significant metabolic benefits over time.

Nutrition and dietary choices are essential factors influencing metabolism. Consuming a balanced diet rich in whole foods, lean proteins, healthy fats, and complex carbohydrates can enhance metabolic efficiency. Additionally, mindful eating techniques—such as paying attention to hunger cues and avoiding distractions during meals—can help individuals develop a healthier relationship with food. This awareness not only supports weight loss efforts but also fosters long-term sustainable eating habits essential for maintaining weight management.

Lastly, lifestyle factors such as sleep quality and stress management are vital for a healthy metabolism. Chronic sleep deprivation can disrupt hormonal balance, leading to increased appetite and cravings, while high stress levels can trigger emotional eating. Prioritizing restful sleep and implementing stress-reduction techniques, such as yoga or meditation, can be instrumental in creating an optimal environment for metabolism to thrive. By understanding these interconnected factors, individuals can develop a holistic approach to weight management that aligns with their unique life stages and personal goals.

Foods and Supplements That Boost Metabolism

Foods and supplements that can boost metabolism play a vital role in achieving and maintaining a healthy weight. Understanding how these elements interact with the body's metabolic processes can empower individuals to make informed dietary choices. For women navigating various life stages, such as menopause or pregnancy, and for adults looking to shed pounds, incorporating specific foods into their diets can provide the necessary support for metabolic health. This chapter will explore effective options that can enhance metabolic rates, helping to create a sustainable approach to weight management.

Protein-rich foods are essential for boosting metabolism due to their high thermic effect, which refers to the energy required for digestion, absorption, and disposal of nutrients. Including lean meats, fish, eggs, legumes, and dairy products in your meals can significantly enhance calorie expenditure. Moreover, protein helps build and maintain muscle mass, which is crucial for a higher resting metabolic rate. For busy professionals and new parents with limited time, meal-prepping protein-packed snacks, such as Greek yogurt or hard-boiled eggs, can be an easy way to support metabolism while managing a hectic schedule.

In addition to protein, incorporating certain spices and herbs can also provide a metabolic boost. Ingredients like cayenne pepper, ginger, and cinnamon have been shown to increase thermogenesis, the process by which the body generates heat and burns calories. Adding these spices to meals not only enhances flavor but also contributes to a more efficient metabolism. Fitness enthusiasts can benefit from experimenting with these flavor enhancers in their cooking, making healthy meals more exciting while reaping the rewards for weight management.

Supplements can also play a supportive role in boosting metabolism, especially for individuals who may struggle to meet their nutritional needs through food alone. Green tea extract, for example, contains catechins that may enhance fat oxidation and improve metabolic rate. Similarly, caffeine is known to stimulate metabolic processes and can be found in various forms, including coffee and certain supplements. However, it is essential for individuals, especially those with health conditions or sensitivities, to consult with healthcare professionals before starting any new supplement regimen.

Lastly, hydration is often overlooked but is a crucial component of a well-functioning metabolism. Water plays a vital role in metabolic processes and can help in calorie burning. Studies suggest that drinking cold water may temporarily boost metabolism as the body expends energy to warm the water to body temperature. For those managing weight, incorporating adequate hydration into their daily routine can enhance metabolic efficiency. By prioritizing water intake alongside a balanced diet rich in metabolism-boosting foods and appropriate supplements, individuals can create a holistic approach to sustainable weight management.

Incorporating High-Intensity Interval Training (HIIT)

Incorporating High-Intensity Interval Training (HIIT) into your fitness routine can be a game changer for weight management, especially for women navigating various life stages. HIIT involves alternating short bursts of intense exercise with periods of rest or lower-intensity activity. This approach not only maximizes calorie burn during workouts but also stimulates post-exercise calorie expenditure, which can be particularly beneficial for those aiming to lose weight. For busy professionals and new parents, HIIT offers a time-efficient solution, allowing you to achieve substantial fitness benefits in as little as 20 to 30 minutes.

One of the significant advantages of HIIT is its adaptability to different fitness levels and personal circumstances. Whether you are a fitness enthusiast or a beginner, HIIT can be tailored to suit your capabilities. For instance, during pregnancy or menopause, you can modify exercises to accommodate your body's changing needs while still reaping the rewards of high-intensity workouts. This flexibility makes HIIT accessible for everyone, including seniors or individuals with health conditions, who can focus on low-impact variations that still elevate heart rates and improve overall fitness.

Integrating HIIT into your routine doesn't have to be complex or require a gym membership. Many effective HIIT workouts can be performed at home with minimal or no equipment. Bodyweight exercises like squats, lunges, and push-ups can be combined with cardio bursts such as jumping jacks or high knees. This home workout option is particularly appealing for those managing tight schedules or looking to create a workout environment that suits their personal preferences. The convenience of home workouts aligns perfectly with sustainable weight management strategies, making it easier to stick to your fitness goals.

To enhance the effectiveness of HIIT, pairing it with mindful eating techniques can yield lasting results. The heightened metabolic activity from HIIT can complement a balanced diet rich in nutrients, supporting not only weight loss but also overall health. Focus on incorporating whole foods, lean proteins, and healthy fats into your meals, and watch how your body responds positively to this combination. By fostering a deeper awareness of food choices and portion sizes, you can create a harmonious balance that supports your weight loss journey.

Finally, building a support system can amplify the benefits of HIIT and overall fitness efforts. Surrounding yourself with like-minded individuals who share similar goals can provide motivation and accountability. Whether it's joining a local fitness group, participating in online forums, or engaging with friends and family, having a network of support can make all the difference. Remember that the journey to permanent weight loss is not just about individual effort; it's about creating an environment that fosters success through encouragement, shared experiences, and collective growth.

Chapter 11: Debunking Weight Loss Myths

Common Myths and Misconceptions

Weight loss is often surrounded by a web of myths and misconceptions that can hinder progress and lead to frustration. Many women, particularly those navigating different life stages such as menopause or pregnancy, may find themselves bombarded with advice that is either misleading or overly simplistic. One common myth is that all calories are created equal, which overlooks the importance of nutrient quality.

While calorie counting is a useful tool, it is vital to understand that the source of those calories—whether they come from whole foods or processed snacks—can significantly impact metabolism, satiety, and overall health.

Another prevalent misconception is the idea that drastic calorie restriction is the key to rapid weight loss. This approach can lead to a cycle of deprivation followed by binge eating, ultimately resulting in weight regain. Instead, sustainable weight management is best achieved through balanced meal planning and moderation. Incorporating a variety of nutrient-dense foods not only supports weight loss but also provides essential vitamins and minerals that the body needs, especially during significant life changes such as pregnancy or menopause when nutritional needs evolve.

The belief that exercise alone is sufficient for weight loss is yet another myth that deserves scrutiny. While physical activity is crucial for burning calories and improving overall health, it is equally important to focus on nutrition. Many busy professionals and new parents struggle to find time for exercise, leading to the false assumption that they cannot lose weight without it. However, integrating mindful eating techniques and making conscious food choices can yield significant results, even without a rigorous workout regimen. This approach emphasizes the importance of creating a balanced lifestyle rather than solely relying on exercise.

Additionally, misconceptions about the role of metabolism can create confusion. Many people believe that they have a "slow metabolism" that prevents them from losing weight, but this may not be entirely accurate. Metabolism can be influenced by factors such as age, muscle mass, and activity level. Advanced metabolism-boosting techniques, such as strength training and proper hydration, can enhance metabolic function. Seniors and individuals with health conditions should focus on strategies tailored to their needs, rather than accepting a fixed notion of metabolism that limits their potential.

Finally, emotional eating is often misunderstood, with many believing that it is simply a lack of willpower. In reality, emotional eating is a complex behavior linked to various psychological and social factors. Overcoming emotional eating requires a deeper understanding of triggers and developing healthier coping mechanisms. Building a support system and seeking guidance from professionals can be invaluable in addressing these behaviors. By debunking these myths and focusing on evidence-based strategies, individuals can cultivate a more effective and sustainable approach to weight management that aligns with their unique goals and circumstances.

Facts Versus Fiction in Weight Loss

In the realm of weight loss, the line between facts and fiction is often blurred, leading to confusion among those seeking effective strategies for managing their weight. Many myths persist, perpetuated by anecdotal evidence, social media influencers, and even well-meaning friends. Understanding what is rooted in scientific evidence versus what is merely a trend can empower individuals to make informed choices about their weight loss journeys. This clarity is especially crucial for women navigating various life stages, busy professionals balancing multiple responsibilities, and health-conscious individuals committed to sustainable changes.

One prevalent myth is the idea that all calories are equal, which oversimplifies the complex nature of nutrition. While calories do matter in terms of energy balance, the source of these calories plays a significant role in weight management. Nutrient-dense foods—such as fruits, vegetables, whole grains, and lean proteins—provide essential vitamins and minerals, aiding in overall health and satiety. In contrast, empty calories from sugary snacks and processed foods can lead to weight gain and health issues, despite being lower in caloric content.

Recognizing this distinction can help individuals make better dietary choices that support lasting weight loss.

Another common misconception is the notion that exercise alone is sufficient for weight loss. While physical activity is a vital component of any weight loss strategy, it is not the sole factor. The relationship between nutrition and exercise is synergistic; without a balanced diet, the results from workouts may be minimal or non-existent. For busy professionals or new parents with limited time, integrating home workouts with mindful eating techniques can create a sustainable approach to weight management. Understanding this interplay allows individuals to tailor their weight loss strategies effectively.

The idea that certain foods can "boost" metabolism or lead to significant weight loss is another area rife with misinformation. Many claims surrounding fat-burning foods lack substantial scientific support. While some foods may have a slight thermogenic effect, the overall impact on weight loss is minimal unless combined with a well-rounded diet and regular exercise.

This myth can lead to frustration and disappointment, especially among those who are eager to find quick fixes. Instead, a focus on holistic health practices, including adequate sleep and stress management, is more effective for achieving and maintaining a healthy weight.

Finally, the belief that weight loss should occur quickly and drastically can set individuals up for failure. Sustainable weight loss is typically gradual, involving lifestyle changes rather than restrictive diets or extreme measures. Emphasizing the importance of patience and consistency can help shift the mindset from seeking immediate results to valuing long-term health. By debunking these common myths and providing evidence-based insights, individuals can create personalized strategies that align with their unique goals, ultimately leading to permanent weight loss and improved well-being.

Expert Insights on Effective Strategies

Effective weight management requires a multifaceted approach that incorporates insights from various experts in the fitness and health industries. These insights emphasize the importance of creating a personalized strategy tailored to individual needs, which can be particularly beneficial for women navigating different life stages, busy professionals, and health-conscious individuals alike. Tailoring fitness regimens and meal plans to suit personal preferences and lifestyles can lead to more sustainable weight loss outcomes, as individuals are more likely to adhere to a program that resonates with their unique circumstances.

Sustainable meal planning is a cornerstone of effective weight management. Experts recommend building a meal plan that incorporates a variety of whole foods, focusing on nutrient-dense options that promote satiety. For busy professionals and new parents, meal prepping can be a game-changer. Setting aside time each week to prepare balanced meals not only saves time during hectic days but also reduces the temptation to resort to unhealthy convenience foods.

Engaging in mindful eating techniques, such as savoring each bite and listening to hunger cues, can further enhance the effectiveness of these meal plans, fostering a healthier relationship with food.

Physical activity plays a crucial role in weight loss and maintenance, and home workouts offer a practical solution for individuals with tight schedules. Fitness experts stress the importance of finding enjoyable forms of exercise that can be easily integrated into daily routines. Whether it's a quick high-intensity interval training session or a calming yoga practice, the key is consistency. Incorporating short bursts of activity throughout the day can also help combat the sedentary lifestyle prevalent in many professions. This approach not only aids in weight management but also contributes to overall well-being.

Overcoming emotional eating is another critical aspect of effective weight management. Experts suggest identifying triggers and developing coping strategies that do not involve food. Techniques such as journaling, meditation, or engaging in hobbies can provide healthy outlets for stress and emotional challenges.

Additionally, building a support system—whether through friends, family, or online communities—can offer encouragement and accountability, making it easier to navigate the ups and downs of the weight loss journey.

Finally, the role of sleep in weight loss is often underestimated. Research shows that inadequate sleep can disrupt hormonal balance, leading to increased cravings and reduced motivation for physical activity. Experts advise prioritizing sleep hygiene to foster better rest, which in turn supports weight management efforts. By integrating these insights into their weight loss strategies, individuals can create a holistic approach that addresses the physical, emotional, and psychological facets of their journey toward permanent weight loss.

Chapter 12: Tailoring Fitness Regimens for Individual Goals

Assessing Personal Fitness Levels

Assessing personal fitness levels is a crucial starting point for anyone embarking on a weight loss journey, particularly for women navigating various life stages. Understanding where you currently stand in terms of physical fitness allows you to set realistic and achievable goals. This assessment can include evaluating your cardiovascular endurance, muscular strength, flexibility, and body composition.

For instance, engaging in a simple fitness test, such as a timed walk or the number of push-ups you can perform in a minute, can provide valuable insights into your current fitness status.

Knowing your baseline helps in creating a personalized plan that accommodates your unique health needs and lifestyle.

For busy professionals and new parents, time constraints can make it challenging to focus on fitness. However, it's essential to prioritize this assessment to ensure that any fitness routine you embark on is effective. Consider utilizing short, efficient workouts that fit into your schedule while still allowing you to monitor your progress. This can involve tracking changes in your endurance over time or noticing improvements in how you feel during everyday activities. Regularly reassessing your fitness levels can help maintain motivation and make necessary adjustments to your routine.

Health-conscious individuals and seniors must also take special care in assessing personal fitness levels. As we age, our bodies undergo various changes that can impact strength, flexibility, and overall stamina. Incorporating balance and flexibility assessments can be especially beneficial for seniors to prevent injuries and maintain independence. Meanwhile, adults with health conditions should consult with healthcare professionals to tailor their fitness assessments appropriately, ensuring that they engage in safe and effective exercises that promote weight loss without compromising their health.

Athletes and fitness enthusiasts may find it beneficial to assess their levels through more advanced metrics, such as VO2 max tests or body fat percentage measurements. These assessments provide a deeper understanding of your physiological capacities and can inform more specialized training programs. However, it's crucial to remember that even for those at a higher fitness level, maintaining a focus on personal progress is key. Establishing personal benchmarks and celebrating small victories can help sustain motivation and commitment.

Lastly, integrating nutrition into your fitness assessment is vital for sustainable weight management. Understanding how your body responds to different foods and meal timing can enhance your overall fitness regimen. Mindful eating practices can help you make more informed decisions regarding your diet, complementing your physical activities. By assessing both your fitness levels and nutritional habits, you create a holistic approach to weight loss that not only fosters immediate results but also supports long-term health and well-being.

Adapting Workouts for Different Life Stages

Adapting workout routines to align with different life stages is essential for women managing their weight effectively. Each phase, from pregnancy to menopause, presents unique physical and hormonal changes that influence both energy levels and exercise capacity. Understanding how these changes affect the body enables more tailored fitness approaches that can promote sustainable weight management and overall well-being. For instance, during pregnancy, engaging in low-impact exercises like walking or swimming can help maintain fitness without unnecessary strain, while postpartum adjustments might include gradually reintroducing strength training to rebuild core stability and muscle tone.

For women experiencing menopause, hormonal fluctuations can lead to weight gain, particularly around the abdomen. Incorporating strength training into workouts becomes increasingly important during this phase, as it not only helps mitigate muscle loss but also boosts metabolism. Additionally, cardiovascular exercises, such as cycling or brisk walking, can support heart health and aid in weight management.

Women in this stage must focus on exercises that enhance bone density and overall strength, thereby addressing the long-term health implications associated with menopause.

Busy professionals often struggle with time constraints, which can hinder the ability to maintain a consistent workout routine. Adapting workouts for this demographic involves focusing on high-intensity interval training (HIIT) and incorporating shorter, more effective sessions that maximize benefits in a limited time. These workouts can be performed at home or in a gym setting and can be adjusted to fit into a packed schedule. Emphasizing the importance of planning and prioritizing fitness can lead to sustainable weight loss outcomes, even amidst a hectic lifestyle.

New parents face the challenge of balancing fitness with childcare responsibilities. Workouts that can be done at home, using body weight or minimal equipment, offer flexibility and convenience. Incorporating the baby into workouts, such as using a stroller for walks or performing exercises while the baby is napping, can help new parents stay active without sacrificing family time. This group needs to set realistic fitness goals and allow for gradual progress, nurturing both physical health and emotional well-being.

Seniors and individuals with health conditions require specialized adaptations to their exercise routines. Focus should be placed on low-impact activities that enhance mobility, flexibility, and strength while minimizing the risk of injury. Activities such as yoga, tai chi, and water aerobics are excellent options that promote overall health while catering to specific limitations. Ensuring that fitness regimens align with personal health goals and physical capabilities enables this demographic to achieve sustainable weight management while improving quality of life. By recognizing the unique needs of each life stage, women can craft effective workout strategies that support long-term health and weight loss success.

Creating a Long-Term Fitness Plan

Creating a long-term fitness plan is essential for anyone looking to achieve sustainable weight loss and maintain a healthy lifestyle. This plan should be tailored to individual needs, taking into consideration factors such as age, fitness level, life stage, and personal preferences. A well-structured fitness plan will not only help in shedding pounds but also promote overall well-being, enhancing both physical and mental health. It is crucial to remember that a long-term approach is about consistency and adaptability rather than quick fixes.

To begin crafting a long-term fitness plan, it is essential to set realistic and achievable goals. These goals should be specific, measurable, attainable, relevant, and time-bound (SMART). For example, instead of stating a vague goal like "I want to lose weight," a SMART goal would be "I aim to lose 10 pounds in three months by exercising three times a week and following a balanced diet." Establishing clear goals helps create a sense of direction and purpose, allowing individuals to track their progress and make necessary adjustments along the way.

Incorporating a variety of workouts into the fitness plan is vital for sustained engagement and effectiveness. This could include a mix of cardiovascular exercises, strength training, flexibility workouts, and activities that promote balance. For busy professionals or new parents, home workouts can be a convenient solution; even short, high-intensity interval training (HIIT) sessions can yield significant results. Additionally, seeking out enjoyable activities, such as dance classes or outdoor sports, can make exercising a more pleasurable experience, ensuring that individuals are more likely to stick with their routines.

Nutrition plays a pivotal role in any long-term fitness plan, and integrating sustainable meal planning is key to achieving lasting weight loss. Developing a balanced diet that includes a variety of whole foods, lean proteins, healthy fats, and plenty of fruits and vegetables can provide the necessary nutrients for both energy and recovery. Mindful eating techniques, such as paying attention to hunger cues and savoring each bite, can help combat emotional eating and promote healthier food choices. Establishing a weekly meal prep routine can also simplify the process, making it easier to stay on track with nutrition goals.

Lastly, building a support system is critical for maintaining motivation and accountability in any long-term fitness journey. This can involve enlisting the help of friends, and family, or joining local fitness groups or online communities. Sharing experiences, challenges, and successes with others can create a sense of camaraderie and encouragement. Additionally, seeking guidance from fitness professionals or nutritionists can provide valuable insights tailored to individual needs, helping to navigate potential obstacles and foster a positive mindset towards achieving and maintaining weight loss goals.

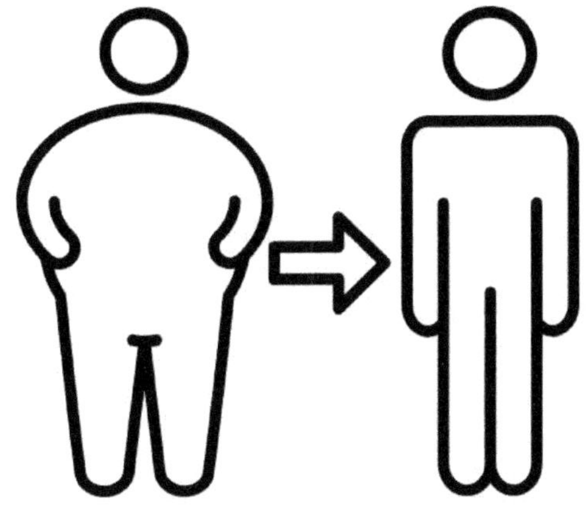

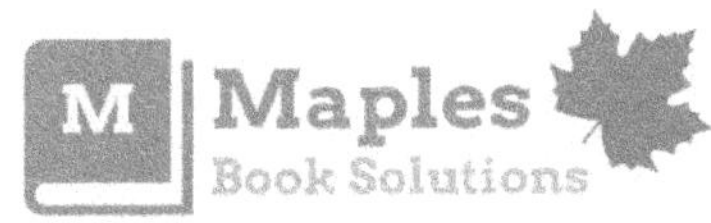

Enjoyed this book?

Positive reviews from awesome customers like you help others to feel confident about choosing Maples Book Solutions too.

Could you take **60 seconds** to go to Amazon platform and share your happy experiences?

We will be forever grateful. Thank you in advance for helping us out!